REAL RECOVERY

REAL RECOVERY:

Healing from Medical Illness And Diagnosis

MICHAEL R. MITCHELL, PHD, LMFT, MAC, CAP

Xulon Press
2301 Lucien Way #415
Maitland, FL 32751
407.339.4217
www.xulonpress.com

Printed in the United States of America.

ISBN-13: 978-1-63221-551-2

TABLE OF CONTENTS

Acronym: **R.E.A.L.**—a working definition.
What is it?
Rehabilitation for whom?

Getting **REA**L Personal: Sharing life experience and spiritual journey—THE QUILT LAYER
AND FABRIC

Physical–Brain-Body Dynamics

CRITICAL (PAIN, SUPPORT TEAM)
INITIAL STAGE OF GRIEF AND LOSS

TRUST FACTORS, ACCEPTING
MEDICAL CARE

RESOLVING EMOTIONAL CONFLICT,
RELEASING RESENTMENT,

RECONCILIATION, RENEWED VALUES, AND
FINDING NEW MEANING IN LIFE

DR. KUBLER- ROSS, **"STAGES OF GRIEF"**:
Replace Denial as the full impact of diagnosis sinks in.

Trials and Tribulations… Early Memories of Faith in
Action (A Personal Reflection)

INTRODUCTION

REAL RECOVERY

RECOGNIZE & REALIZE REALITY

EXPECT CHANGE.TIME VARIANCE
"THIS TOO SHALL PASS"

ACCEPT LIMITATIONS, FAILURE,
FATIGUE & GUILT

LIVE LIFE ON PURPOSE, WITH
INTENTION AND MINDFULNESS.
PRACTICE FOR TOTAL HEALING AND A
NATURAL STATE OF CALMNESS. AIM FOR
WHOLENESS IN BODY, MIND, AND SOUL/
TOTAL MIND-BODY AWARENESS IN THE
PRESENT, ABSENT OF JUDGEMENT.

FULFILL YOUR DESTINY: YOUR
FOOTSTEPS IN THE SAND

FAITH IN AN UNCERTAIN TIME AND PLACE

The most important point I wish to impart upon my readers is the following: Rehabilitation is a choice. One can will themselves to health and wellness!

Furthermore, this book is not particularly written to address those of any particular religious persuasion or orientation. It is, however, for the benefit of those in the faith communities who wish to gain a deeper appreciation for the writer's personal history as a Christian with regards to the importance and value of positive belief, the infinite possibilities of medical miracles, healing power, and the transformation of the mind in order to will oneself to better health, peace, and joy. One may do this by living life on purpose, with mindfulness practice towards recovery and ultimate restoration. Most importantly, this writer acknowledges that

FAITH is a universal resource available to all who are receptive to the belief in the power of supernatural healing through faith.

Whether you are reading this book out of intellectual curiosity or because you or someone close to you is in need of a resource to help them take life to the next level of optimal functioning, I hope that you will approach the subject matter with an open heart and mind. As a clinical therapist, I am often found guilty of over-explaining when it comes to the subject of healing and recovery from mental and physical affliction. Perhaps my years of clinical training in behavioral health and marriage and family therapy have motivated within me a sense of urgency, given the status of the broken family and marital systems in America. I feel that it may be a dis- service to not speak on a topic for which I have the utmost respect and personal obligation to share with you.

First I must digress for a moment to give attention to what is perhaps one of the worst devastating pandemic our global society has witnessed in centuries: COVID-19, also known as the novel coronavirus. Many lives have been impacted, and still as this book comes off the press unknown numbers are unaccounted for. Survivors' lives will be changed, and the emotional toll cannot be calculated or fully comprehended. We can be appreciative of modern technology, especially mass media for information, however disseminated or reliable in order to increase survival through education and self-advocacy.

The ideas expressed in this book are intended to educate, stimulate, and inspire any person who has struggled with a medical condition or illness which may render one incapacitated or with a desire to resume normal life as experienced in past. When you finish this book, you may be truly convinced that you have a choice, that you can direct your life towards wholeness. This writer is suggesting to you that there is an adventure in healing, and that this change comes from new insight, changed feelings, and new behaviors. With a "walk of faith," you may experience a miracle. Each section of this book represents the various personal trials this writer and perhaps most individuals may relate to in their struggles towards genuine health and wholeness, to avoid intense suffering. The hope is that you, the reader, gain a greater appreciation for how positive change can happen with hope and faith, when one is deeply aware of reality. As a bonus, it can be used as a self-help guide with practical tools for spiritual intervention. Finally, this book is intended to help the reader understand and embrace the idea that miracles of healing and restoration are manifested through faith and conviction.

Getting Personal:

As with many of my public speaking engagements, presentations, and workshops, I feel compelled to maintain ethical disclosure and inform you, the reader, that this material is based on my personal and professional experience and in no way serves to advise medical information, treatment, or recommendations. You should always consult your healthcare provider when considering treatment for your medical or health needs. It is also important that you or a loved one seriously considers how to embrace specific medical and lifestyle concerns and begin to reconstruct a plan that works for your unique needs.

This book is designed to share personal and anecdotal accounts of real life situations which will hopefully keep you engaged in the conversation and study of how to apply helpful and practical life-sustaining tools in the process of regaining total life balance after being diagnosed with a medical or health-related challenge.

I can recall many instances in my clinical practice where a married couple would present with stress related to one individual's major medical issues and the other spouse/partner might exhibit stressful emotions and psychological symptoms as if they had the medical condition themselves. This is not uncommon in the human experience. Actually, there is a known phenomenon that is identified as "secondary trauma", which is sometimes crippling to first responders as a result of the victims they rescue and serve. Even therapists such as myself can be in denial of the impact of years of working in a profession that has its "casualties."

In my years of clinical practice, I have come to the awareness of chronological age and one's stage of life. Over the years I have observed that many men and, most recently, women who have been in the work force for decades find it difficult to embrace the notion of retirement or "job loss." From my perspective, much of these prevailing dynamics may stem from personality type such as the "Type A workaholic." This may also be described as a person who is driven towards success and achievement. Not only does the individual present with symptoms of depression, sadness, anxiety, and overwhelming grief, but their adjustment or lack thereof appears to have an impact on family, loved ones, and friends.

The disappointment in many lives occurs when people lose their identity and authentic selves to defined roles and titles. This seems to hinder their ability to rebound from life's unfortunate circumstances, catastrophic illness, and unforeseen setbacks.

An important point that I want my readers to take away from this book is that life is paralyzing when struggles surround us, but there is no shame in being still. Even in ancient history we can learn that there is value in slowing down the soul to make each day matter as life permits.

MANY PEOPLE, OUT OF HABIT, NEVER SLOW DOWN THE PACE OF THEIR LIVES UNTIL THEY ARE FORCED TO DO SO.

They get ill, experience an accident, or lose their job and/ or income suddenly, and they have no choice but to reduce their speed and change their normal routine. Most of the time this process lends itself to positive results, even if the person initially resisted their required rest periods, rehabilitation, and therapy. This is an incredible opportunity for daily devotion and positive affirmations, because it lends itself to supernatural intervention. This may lead us to develop a sense that simply being present, being mindful, trusting in the process, and resting assured of God's goodness is our priority. The tranquility of opening the window to peace of mind brings peace and calm. Learning to let go and release with little faith will multiply the supernatural healing of body and soul.

Please allow me to share with you a brief personal event that changed my life on the exact date of January 16, 2020. On the night before, I found myself alone in bed and attempted to rise from prone position to go to the bathroom, only to fall hard onto the floor in a horizontal position. Unable to maneuver to a better position to bear my weight, my survival instincts automatically sent a message to my brain to elevate for balance and mobility. The problem with this directive from the command center of the brain was that the neurotransmitters were not firing or responding in unison with my muscles in order to accomplish the desired task. I actually attempted to pull myself up from the floor using the foot rail bed post, but my left side was completely inept, rendering a totally limp grasp to no avail. The right side attempted to compensate, but those muscles were also impaired. Hence, I found myself struggling and scooting in a backward position toward the lower furniture, unaware of the numerous scratches and bruises sustained on both arms from the wood floor.

A loud but bold cry came out of my mouth, which was a plea to God for help. I clearly remember asking God for the strength to be able to rest on my knees so that I would be able to humbly pray for strength and power. Tears flowed from my eyes while I had a serious talk with my Lord and Savior. I looked up to the heavens with tearful eyes and prayed for rest from this struggle for safety and survival. In hindsight I recall lying in the bed, nothing short of a miracle, passing out, and totally resting for at least thirty minutes. I say that only a miracle would have placed my body in bed because when I finally awakened and attempted to search for my two cell phones in bed (personal and work), realized that I could not operate either because I was unable to grip them. They would fall constantly, and even if

I tried to dial numbers, my brain would not execute the functions successfully.

Finally realizing that this was a traumatic medical situation, my brain denied me the ability to have rational thought. I proceeded to take my daily shower while still wearing my house slippers. I still believe that the brain is a remarkable creation from God, superior by far to any artificial intelligence or computer.

Researchers have found that there are automatic pathways that execute behaviors and habits, and because of the brain's plasticity, it is possible to compensate for loss of cell function. I am reminded of our habits, daily activities like grooming and dressing skills. After I left the shower, I discovered that I could only dry myself with one hand; the task of dressing was a real challenge. Out of habit, I always prepare and arrange my attire for work the night before. This simplified my morning, but the real struggle was attempting to dress myself. There was real perspiration in this process, and I looked in the mirror and discovered that even a preschool toddler could be more proficient in self-dressing.

Keep in mind if you will, I actually felt normal as I pressed down on my garments. I concealed the fact that I had no belt with a vest and carried on. Isn't this indicative of how we are blind to our dysfunction in our daily lives? To make matters worse, I grabbed my keys, personal bag, and wallet, only to later discover that my bag was left on the sidewalk near my vehicle (it was later returned to me). Unable to set the alarm system, I rushed to my auto. Again, this was a daily routine, so I began my journey and something in my mind (perhaps rational) directed my path toward the local community hospital only fifteen minutes away. As you may surmise from this scenario, I was not in any position to drive my vehicle, which resulted in a traffic collision and emergency paramedics having to extricate me from my vehicle and transport me to a regional hospital where I would lie in the emergency room and udnergo extensive evaluation and observation for a medical diagnosis of CVA/ stroke with hemiparesis.

I am forever reminded of the notion of faith in action, because how you work through your situation is determined by your belief and trust in the miracle of healing in spite of the physical and emotional pain one may endure. This book is designed

to guide you through the crucial stages and pro-
gression of recovery.

THE THREE PHASES OF RECOVERY

FAITH

PHASE ONE

Whether you or someone you know who has been diagnosed with a medical condition and treated for the first time has a pre-existing diagnosis or co-occurring (multiple) medical or psychiatric conditions, one should always be take into consideration many factors in providing the necessary care and appropriate treatment for the best standard of care.

First of all, finding the necessary support system is essential. You may do so by providing your health care provider with the names and contacts of individuals that you consent to discuss and advocate in your best interest.

My personal experience was "God sent," because I have a spouse who was available 24/7 and remained at my bedside whether in-patient hospitalization or at discharge to home. As a patient and in recovery or home rehabilitation, you have to rely on family, friends, and significant support in order to communicate, translate and exchange information between medical professionals and you, the patient. There were many times my comprehension or ability to communicate were altered by my medical condition.

In this stage it is also important to have available insurance policies, medical and healthcare history, the name of one's employer, and contact phone numbers. Keeping in mind the HIPPA and Protective Health Information (PHI) ACT, you must have the legal means of exchanging information solely for your ability to consider Disability benefits and Family Leave (FMLA) benefits. It is not a requirement to release your medical records for your legal protection, but you may consider requesting a letter of documentation for work.

Based on my prior experience as a Behavioral Healthcare provider and patient, I have come to realize that it can be rather disheartening and demoralizing to receive a rejection or denial letter from insurance companies when it comes to your health care and disability benefits. I will elaborate more on this subject later as we explore readiness stages of function.

When someone has been immobilized and confined to a bed with limited movement, or perhaps in isolation in the critical stage of illness, they may experience sensory deprivation. Their sensory input may have been altered, especially with regard to vision, tactile response (touch), smell (the olfactory system), and taste. These problems were consistent in my case, and ultimately contributed to an increase in moodiness and irritability. Subsequently, it may increase a sense of helplessness and feelings of hopelessness.

Keep in perspective that firstly there are natural changes that one will undergo, which will impact self-care, nutrition, and overall health during the various stages of illness. Simple skills are the essential building blocks to higher level function. I have a personal philosophy which I am reminded to share with you because I hold this belief in my heart and soul:

"Little by little, one goes far."

In other words, take "baby steps" towards your progress in recovery.

Even at the early stages of recovery, one can practice mindful meditation and prayer. There will be a section later on the subject of meditation and prayer along with important spiritual affirmations.

Mindful meditation was reported to have originated from Eastern spiritual thought and is now considered an evidence-based science that has shown positive correlation with the reduction of pain and inflammation, as well as an increase in immune function. While the person suffering from a medical condition may experience isolation and depressive feelings, this practice and prayer can aid in refocusing attention by "reframing" that feeling of lacking control to more strength, based in incremental steps over a period of time in both intensity and duration.

HOPE

PHASE TWO

I prefer to relate to Phase Two as a middle stage, if you will, because it basically means that you or your loved one has already been informed of the medical diagnoses and perhaps some treatment options, as well as a tentative prognosis of the condition. It does not necessarily mean that you are out of a critical stage or have completely recovered from the identified medical condition. Ideally you are in a better position, cognitively, to gather more information in order to comprehend and possibly speak to your care team, consisting of medical doctors, specialists, nurses, rehabilitation providers and family member/significant other(s).

I find it necessary to share an important and relevant perspective which I would like to borrow from the addiction recovery community, which lends itself to anyone who finds themselves in a state of brokenness and life disruption as a result of a health or medical condition. This SERENITY PRAYER can sum up the beginning of a new manner of cognitive and spiritual processing:

"GOD, GRANT ME THE SERENITY TO ACCEPT THE THINGS I CANNOT CHANGE: COURAGE TO CHANGE THE THINGS I CAN: AND THE WISDOM TO KNOW THE DIFFFERENCE."

This well-known prayer continues with deep religious and biblical references; however, it is my intention that this message alone gives rise to the understanding that the reflection of spiritual connections can catapult you to a new trajectory of life and purpose, even as you question your own mortality.

After the initial stage of recuperation, there are natural changes that you the patient may undergo which will affect your attention and awareness. This will impact your self-care, nutrition, and overall health during various stages of you recovery. Emotionally, you (the patient) may find yourself consumed with feelings about family, friends, and professional (co-worker) relationships.

I can recall the countless stories of patients and clients that I have counseled over the past decades, many of whom were individuals and couples dealing with medical issues such as infertility, heart disease, diabetes, gastrointestinal issues, hypertension, and the like. The reality is that some unknown, unanticipated, and often times unwanted medical conditions change the trajectory of people's lives to the extent that they not only alter their present and future plans but may also be viewed as inconvenient and impact their spiritual lives as never before.

This amazing aspect of therapeutic intervention is that everyone has a personal journey, and when you share your narrative and your "truth" you will find a reason to shift and reframe your thinking towards HOPE and begin to make choices which can lead to miracles, recovery, and unknown blessings even while you may be on the verge of hopelessness and helplessness. This is why I appreciate the adage "Let go and let God." I can attest to the spiritual healing in families and relationships impacted by medical and health challenges. The idea of replacing hurt and fear with trust and hope is an ultimate sacrifice and commitment.

The middle phase of recovery is an important time to not only focus on your overall medical situation but your attitude as well. Recognizing the fact that you are not able to resume your normal life routine may cause you to feel annoyed with the process of healing over time. My week of inpatient hospitalization seemed more like a month as I literally stood by the door with a cane, walker, and chair, waiting to be discharged. A diagnosis and prognosis is foreign to one who is anxious to get back to the familiar. We forget that even in prayer man's time is not the same as God's plan for your right time. This has to be kept in perspective if you are going to successfully heal and prosper.

AS you become more aware of your surroundings and reflect on your perceived losses, you may question loved ones who were at your bedside, in your home, on the telephone with you, or making contact to offer words of care and support. You may have conflicting feelings of anger, betrayal, and a sense of abandonment. I must admit that I found myself consumed with all of these emotions, as I received deliveries of flowers and phone calls, in addition to face-to-face bedside visit while in the emergency room. My wonderful sisters from my church prayed with me, and I will forever be grateful for their support because they traveled for many miles just to support me at a most critical time. Those who make promises are more than likely to disappoint and bring sorrow in a place of yearning for comfort.

I am introducing a section on the grief process later in this book in order to highlight the importance of deep healing from the heart and soul.

This is a time to attempt to become more organized and structured. Consider using a pocket calendar. With this visual aid, you may find yourself better able to focus and perhaps gain more awareness of your daily engagements. I have also found this to be helpful with the various scheduled visits with medical specialists and rehabilitation therapists (occupational, physical. and speech).

Medical illness may present simultaneously with emotional pain or trauma, as I have previously alluded to from personal and shared accounts from others. Many times a disease such as heart or auto-immune deficiency can appear gradually and or at one unexpected time. These medical conditions may affect sleep patterns, eating, diet, and hydration, along with multiple related medical complications. Secondary and underlying symptoms may have considerable psychological and mental health affects with increased anxiety and depression. From my clinical practice experience, I have found that men in particular have difficulty sharing this information, and once they begin to share this information about their diagnosis, it actually increases anxiety (possibly due to fear of the possibility that recovery may not be quick and easy, but chronic and life-long).

This brings my topic and discussion of REAL RECOVERY to the idea of what it means to not feel in control of one's body. As in my situation dealing with mobility and coordination challenges, as well as neurological, visual, and cognitive deficits, Admitting to fear and other emotions that arise from the unknown, be it a chronic or sudden medical diagnosis, will bring about a series of emotional reactions. Although this book is not intended to deal with the subject of end of life planning, I am mindful of the remarkable contributions of a noted psychiatrist and frequently cited authority on the subject of Grief and Loss. Dr. Elisabeth Kubler-Ross identified the "five stages of grief." Subsequent to her contribution to the field, there have been other contributors with additional stages that perhaps expound on the existential meaning of life and death. For the sake of this book, I hope to stay focused on the primary goal of life and living with maximum joy, purpose, and meaning. I do feel that the stages of grief are relevant in that they can allow us to explore the normal human reaction to real life events that occur which are out of the ordinary, unexpected, unplanned, and even unwantedly catastrophic. It is commonly shared by behaviorists that we humans are not psychologically equipped to immediately accept or even comprehend abnormal life events such as tragedy, death, or loss. According to Dr. Kubler-Ross, the following stages are applicable to this process. I shall guide you through each in a most simplistic manner to help with our understanding of the recovery process:

1. SHOCK, DENIAL, DISBELIEF
2. ANGER
3. BARGINING
4. DEPRESSION
5. ACCEPTANCE

At the time of this book's release, our country (and our world at large) has already faced the loss of countless lives, as well as many diagnosed COVID-19 survivors from the 2020 pandemic, as the media has reported on a daily basis. The prevailing themes of survivors permeate their testimonies of deep philosophical and spiritual healings with resounding gratitude and praise to their God and their personal savior and comforter through crisis.

Perhaps this is the common denominator for us to embrace as a society, with emphasis on medicine for the soul as well as the body.

Facing a "near-death experience" resulting from illness may not necessarily mean that one will experience one or all of the aforementioned stages of grief or loss, but it does give rise to the psychological and emotional factors that may impede one's ability to move through the crisis with renewed spiritual values, acceptance, and sometimes appreciation for having had the opportunity to acquire a personal testimony that can draw others to the need for reconciliation. These testimonies can help others refocus on what is the ultimate will of God in their lives—to heal, restore, deliver, and prove Himself as sovereign, with a plan to preserve and not destroy.

This may also be analogous to other areas of one's life where there are questions not about medical diagnoses, but about financial and economic struggles, loss of relationships, and even divorce. It is only natural to wonder why this situation may have come into one's life. The most important point is how we choose to manage and survive.

Trials and Tribulations are often addressed within the Christian faith. My own personal account is perhaps worthy of sharing, especially since I was raised by Christian parents who were always active in church and worship community. I can recall a vivid personal experience at age ten, after playing a game of baseball with friends on a Saturday afternoon, when a random brawl took place in the neighborhood and a stray bullet struck me in the left side of my neck. I found out later that it actually entered my neck and exited my back. At the onset of this situation I found myself in a traumatized flight reaction as I ran home down the street, bleeding profusely. My mother heard my loud cry, opened the door, and saw the bloody shirt; she was in a panic mode, but a friend who followed me on his bicycle pleaded with her to deliver me by his bicycle to the hospital, less than a quarter mile from where I painfully stood in shock. I remember my friend, William, promising to my mother, "I'll get him there." I cried out "No! I can't!" and my mother insisted that I get on the bicycle, stating that she would be following me. My father was at work at the time, and within minutes my mother was in the emergency room as my clothing was cut from my body while I was being medically stabilized.

In retrospect, I realize that an ambulance was not likely to respond in a timely manner, so my trust in a most unconventional mode of transport was guided by my mother's faith and the love and confidence of another human being, guided by God revealing Himself in what could have been a dire outcome. This is why even today I have developed a deeper faith connection than when I first believed.

GRADITUDE

PHASE THREE

At this point in the recovery process it may seem reasonable, or even logical, that one has moved beyond a "critical stage." You, the patient, have survived to live through the diagnostic experience. This may actually become a crucial point in the recovery process because it opens up new meaning for spiritual connection, life purpose, and the surmising of what it may have taken to process and move beyond the "through." It ought to be a point at which it is a confirmation that faith is not optional, but essential to life.

Upon further review and exploration of the "stages of grief," it is this writer's belief that one cannot fully recover from the effects of a medical illness, diagnosis, or medical condition before the recognition of the human emotions which hinge on health and wellness.

As a mental health professional and behavioral researcher, I have discovered consistently that anger is a normal human emotion. Unfortunately, it is often misconstrued as a pejorative cultural norm. Anger actually has a benefit to human experience because it allows us to express feeling. Anger itself is not necessarily the "enemy" to others. My experience has proven that people have a tendency to avoid this feeling because it may bring about feelings of guilt, shame, and perhaps learned behaviors from childhood parental models where there is an insistence on repression, denial of its existence. Not validating the experience may in fact inspire the opposite negative effect of "acting out" as a function of conflict.

Biblical scholars in the Christian faith have often cited the conversation Jesus Christ had with His father God at the time of His crucifixion:

> *"My God, why have you forsaken me?"*
> *(Matthew 27:46)*

It is believed that Jesus understood that despite speaking against His father, He would be forgiven for His anger; like us, God understands when we are faced with grief and loss.

Two of my most special biblical references to the subject of anger are as follows:

> "Do not let the sun go down on your anger," and "Good sense makes one slow to anger."(Proverbs 19:11)

These prescribed messages have deep meaning and purpose as they pertains to practicing strategies for living a life of hope and transformation.

The writing of this book has a serendipitous reference to my life journey. The very subject of grief affected me personally, as evidenced by the repressed resentment, hurt, sadness, and disappointment that I admittedly harbored during the most critical time of my medical challenge. Family members and "loved ones" made void and empty promises to reach my bedside, only to literally fail to deliver. A sense of isolation by those who made empty promises seemed more pronounced than the wonderful responses from co-workers, friends, and strangers.

"Strangers." I have come to belief that there are no strangers in the world. We are all related in the kingdom of God. I am forever grateful that God keeps His promises at all times and in all places. My church also supported me in my need by showing up to my home and making personal contact with me while praying, especially when I could not pray for myself.

I have learned, and perhaps you may also share similar narratives that are compelling to the experience of faith-based communities and those seeking to find a more fulfilling life of sustained joy and peace. Blood relatives and sometimes extended family and friends may become unaware of the hurt, harm, and negative emotional impact their failed commitments and promises have on those who suffer, as if to add to the burden itself. My plea to you as I encourage myself is to try to understand that this question of faith is to help you to grow spiritually. Therefore ACCEPT the anger, the tears, and simply allow the feelings to flow as a fountain or babbling brook. Eventually you may be able to work through the loss and forgive yourself through the reconciliation inherent in forgiveness of others who disappoint. You are also more prepared to let go of your past losses with renewed hope for a brighter future.

GETTING YOUR HOUSE IN ORDER
By Starting with an Attitude of Gratitude

This well-expressed notion can be summed up to simply speak to the importance of staying vital and victorious over your diagnoses and medical condition. This involves the combination of medical access, mental health, positive support systems, personal hobbies, and healthy habits and practices. I prefer to frame this as intentional living and maintaining a spiritual focus; hence, purposeful living requires honesty and authentic generosity. It is essential to move past hurts by releasing anger, letting go of hurt, and an intentional move towards forgiveness in order to rebuild your life. The idea of practicing mindfulness will allow you to pay more attention to how you not only adjust your physical body and posture with daily exercise, but also begin to observe your inner states and judgements about who you are or how you see yourself on the inside. As we begin to relax and become more introspective, it increases the space for God to reveal Himself in a warm, loving, and empathetic manner:

"Where there is light, the darkness diminishes."

Illumination

It is most important in the recovery process that we pay attention to basic life functions such as breathing, walking, sitting, and even lying down in an effort to improve one's heart rate with regulated restoration and healing for the body. Paying more attention to subtle changes in one's body is the starting point of meditation and positioning oneself in a posture of prayer.

Although I do not claim to be an expert in the practice of mindfulness meditation, I have applied techniques and the experience of yoga, which is another form of meditation aimed at helping one to become more attuned and compassionate. This also helps bring about a sense of peace, allowing us to become more available to others. I have discovered that we have the receptivity to become more kind and patient with other people as well.

Absent of this awareness, it is believed that a person will simply live the same old patterns, often ineffective and dysfunctional. The concept of "slowing down" may seem simplistic, but it is the only way to improve concentration and learning. I have had to apply this principal to my own life, as I experience new ways of resolving problems with new "tools" (like rehabilitation) to improve my way of living. A better way is to explore what it means to have balance.

The principal and practice of mindfulness is useful for activities of daily living (ADL) skills, especially eating, diet, and nutrition. I often encourage myself and others to apply this practice to eating a simple meal, which we often take for granted as an unconscious act. When we do so with intention, we may begin to use our entire God-given faculties such as vision, taste, and smell, along with visualization for the full benefit of human consumption.

An example could be how my meals are often prepared with fresh vegetables, where I can experience the colors and textures and imagine how various food items are grown from the earth with natural nutrients and sources of innate vitamins before they are carefully harvested from the farm to the table and prepared for my body's intake and benefit. This mindful process offers more value and "conscious awareness" while eating that does not take one to the degree of overeating or under-eating, but instead makes one appreciative for the balance and centeredness. In addition, it is beneficial to know that the cells in my body are working towards regeneration and healing, even to the basic physiological level of increased oxygen and blood flow.

In the state of MINDFULNESS there is no judgement or shame, even if it surfaces for a moment in time. This is why we should ALWAYS maintain an "ATTITUDE OF GRADITUDE' on a daily basis.

Fortify your house:

The ultimate goal of THE REAL RECOVERY concept is to equip you with the necessary tools to preserve a peaceful life existence and to use our God-given gifts to draw attention to the expression of praise and gratitude as we exalt the Lord! Increased understanding and knowledge come from the ability to "be still and Know." Psalms 111:10 states:

"The fear of the Lord is the beginning of wisdom."

This message is helpful because the wisdom to discern when to speak, act, or listen is important.

I am not a proponent of making New Year's resolutions, but I can recall during my younger years having responded to the frequently question asked: "What is your New Year's resolution?" I know without a doubt that for a least a decade it was the same response: "Talk less and listen more."

This can be rather challenging for someone in my profession, and I may have not been as consistent in honoring this commitment; however I know that I had and still frequently catch myself going back to a safe place of peace. I "pause" to think, feel, express, and energize a positive mind set

The fact that we "fortify our house" symbolizes gaining the ability to strengthen our creativity, preserve life, and gain a greater sense of autonomy over our worldly affairs. This may include keeping important appointments with medical specialists and rehabilitation.

COMPREHENSIVE SELF-CARE MANAGEMENT

Maintain regular follow-up with your primary care physician regarding new and updated information concerning immunization and respiratory disease; begin to take proactive steps to prevent additional medical complications.

The prescription for total healing comes with mindful discipline and focus. This may mean avoiding negative people, gossip, excessive use of alcohol, media, and other addictions which may numb emotional feelings or delay and inhibit healthy grief and recovery. The following list, although not exhaustive, should be considered:

- Avoid idle time and social isolation.
- Always keep a calendar; make daily plans and activities in advance.

- Get your personal affairs in order (update medical directives, establish a living will, take care of insurance).
- Join a social cause that will impact the lives of other people; boost your immune system through service and kindness to others.
- Get plenty of sleep and rest (8-10 hours daily).
- Maintain a healthy diet and nutrition.
- Set a routine exercise program within medical guidelines for your individual situation.
- Reframe your values about money, the meaning of success, and the "best job."

Finally, focus on productivity and collaborative decision making to maximize good judgement and avoid negative impulses. Planning ahead and utilizing resources gives one a sense of security and protection. Strive to leave a legacy that is sustainable and memorable for the next generation and those that matter to you.

With the aforementioned considerations, we can apply spiritual and mindfulness practice that actually help to develop new pathways in the brain and, on a chemical level, form new perceptions, as well as resolve and take on new actions. We are able to safely confront our inner critical voice and "free up" past hurt, loss, and fear. As in job loss, you may have sadness or negative feelings, but you are better prepared to manage disappointments, upsets, and physical pain as "bumps in the road" rather than end points.

The final contentment through acceptance is taking responsibility for your health, as this book has hopefully demonstrated, for renewed strength and security wherever you are in the moment. Remember the universe has an infinite and abundant supply of healing power for your **REAL RECOVERY**.

DAILY AFFIRMATIONS
AND REFLECTIONS

God will always sustain and keep me when I need strength. (Isaiah 10:31)

I will let go of questioning and begin to trust in the power that is all knowing. (Proverbs 3- 5:6)

My submission to God will lead to greater trust and increase my faith.(James 4:7-8)

My strength and peace will come in a supernatural experience like an eagle that soars. (Isaiah 10:11)

I am grateful for my caring neighbors who are near me. (Proverbs 27:10)

God's infinite wisdom knows what i need right now. (Philippians 4:19)

My future is ordained by God. (Jeremiah 29:11)

My trial is revealed in this struggle for a greater purpose. (Philippians 1:8)

Faith is my anchor when I am discouraged.

My hope is in the unseen and not based on my own understanding.

I am more determined to cooperate with God's inspiration and assistance each day of my life.

I will keep an open door to my heart!

I will learn to encourage myself by responding to God's invitation to a closer relationship in my daily life.

I will remain grateful even in small miracles, like breathing air.

I will meditate on God's word both day and night.

I decree healing in my body and mind continually.

I will bless the Lord at all times and praise Him for the good and bad that befalls me.

I will look to the hills from which cometh my help.

I will be mindful to use my anger to fight for truth, justice, positive healing, and change within me and in the world.

I can do all things through Christ who gives me strength. (Phillippians 4:13)

I am worthy of God's grace. (Isaiah 103:12)

I will listen more and pause before I speak. (James 1:19)

I will get up and do something.

I will press until something happens.

great is Your mercy, O Lord, give me life according to Your promise! (PSALM 119)

God is good all the time!

I will strive to remain humble at all times!

MY PERSONAL JOURNEY/ NOTES

DATE/ TIME ENTRIES

_____

_____

_____

_____

_____

_____

_____

_____

_____

_____

_____

_____

_____

_____

_____

_____

_____

_____

_____

_____

_____

_____

_____

_____

_____

_____

_____

_____

My Personal Journey/ Notes

_____

_____

_____

_____

_____

_____

_____

_____

_____

_____

_____

_____

_____

_____

_____

_____

REFERENCES/ SUGGESTED READING

<u>Death the Final Stage of Growth</u> Elisabeth Kubler-Ross
  Prentice-Hall International Inc.
London 1975

<u>Holy Bible: NKJV New King James Version</u>
  American Bible Society Thomas Nelson, Inc.
New York 1979

<u>The Living Bible Paraphrased</u>
  Tyndale House Publishers, Inc.
Wheaton, Ill. 1971

<u>The Human Brain</u>
  McWittrock, Jackson Beatty, et. Al
  Prentice-Hall Englewood Clifts N.J. 1977

The Brain Dr. David Eagleman
Public Brdocast (PBS) DVD PBS.Org. 2015

Keys to Practicing Mindfulness, Practical Strategies
Manuela Mischke Reeds WW. Norton & Company New York. London 2015

The Purpose Driven Life, Rick Warren
The Purpose Driven Church Zondervan Press 2002

ABOUT THE AUTHOR

Michael R. Mitchell, PhD is a licensed marriage and family therapist in the State of Georgia, a Master Addiction Professional and certified Substance Abuse Professional in the State of Florida. He earned his B.A. in psychology from Pitzer College, Claremont, California, his M.A. in psychology from Washington University in St. Louis, MO, and his PhD. in behavioral health from the International University for Graduate Studies in the English Commonwealth of St. Kitts. Dr. Mitchell is an educator and has worked extensively in hospital settings and community clinics as a mental health professional. He has maintained a private practice for over three decades.

ACKNOWLEDGEMENTS

THIS BOOK IS DEDICATED IN HONOR OF:

THE GLORY OF GOD FOR HIS LASTING GRACE AND MERCIES!

MY SPOUSE AND LIFE PARTNER OF THIRTY YEARS, EZRIA YEARLING, WHO HAS ALWAYS BEEN THERE AS MY SUPPORT

TO OUR PARENTS AND FAMILY MEMBERS, NOW RESTING IN THE ARMS OF THE LORD.

TO MICHAEL CARSON, MY HEART'S INSPIRATION

TO MY MENTOR AND PASTOR, THE REVEREND DR. CYNTHIA L. HALE, AND THE

PRAYER WARRIORS OF THE RAY OF HOPE CHRISTIAN CHURCH OF DECATUR, GEORGIA.

TO MY EARTH ANGELS, ANGELA AND CHERYL, SISTERS IN CHRIST

SPECIAL RECOGNITION AND GRADITUDE TO ALL OF THE COMPETENT REHABILITATION PROFESSIONALS WHO HAVE WORKED ON MY BEHALF FOR BOTH PHYSICAL AND MENTAL RECOVERY.